THE DECAY OF CARING:

TAKING BACK YOUR HEALTHCARE IN AN

IMPERSONAL WORLD

Paul Jurkowski

INDEX

FOREWORD

Decay: (from Merriam-Webster) 1). to decline from a sound or prosperous condition. 2). To decrease, usually gradually in size, quantity, activity, or force. 3). To fall into ruin. 4). To decline in health, strength, or vigor.

I have worked in several healthcare systems in medicine for 37 years, and in psychiatry since I started my residency in 1986, and over the past 25 years I have seen a gradual deterioration in the connection between providers and patients/clients. This deterioration is not specific to any one provider or system, but has occurred as a general change in attitude and values over most of healthcare. If you have seen and felt this happening in your life, please read this book. Even if you haven't, it is vital that everyone understand what is happening in healthcare, as if we don't shift the trends, it almost certainly will get worse.

Throughout this book I have used the word "client" in place of "patient," as the word patient focuses more on the idea of illness instead of the whole person with all of their strengths and desires for their life. "Provider" is used for the people we seek care from, as not all providers are MDs or DOs but come from several backgrounds.

This book is really about you. I've tried to avoid quoting a lot of statistics, research citations, and references, but have focused on the things you don't see when you walk into a providers office, what you will be dealing with, and what you can do to change your visit. If you'd like to get more involved,

join our forum at www.takebackourcare.org

PART ONE: MEDICINE

Chapter One: It Was Always About Money

A little thought and a little kindness are often worth more than a great deal of money.

John Ruskin

Money cannot buy peace of mind. It cannot heal ruptured relationships, or build meaning into a life that has none.

Richard M. DeVos

25 years ago...

In the 1980s a dramatic change in healthcare was beginning to develop. Doctors and hospitals, quite frankly, were charging too much for services. Individuals knew this, and so did corporations and governmental organizations. Medicare itself had started a "Prospective Payment System" that sought to limit the escalating fees for services. Business and organization owners saw increasing costs insuring their employees as well, and they reached a breaking point. Over the following years, companies and organizations would unite to form huge buyer groups which in their combinations had tens of thousands of what they called "lives" to buy coverage for, and began putting pressure on doctors, hospitals, and health insurance companies to provide more care for less money. They received protection in Congress from being prosecuted under anti-kickback laws in 1986, furthering the spread of these buyer groups. This was, at first glance, a much needed change in the healthcare payment system. Had this been a negotiated change, we might have seen a new approach that allowed for a compromise between the profits of business and the needs of its employees and healthcare providers, but instead the buyer groups became so powerful that healthcare providers were forced to not just compromise, but struggle to give increasing amounts of care for less money, or be cut off from much of their payments. Gradually, healthcare providers themselves had to form into groups of providers, or join larger organizations including HMOs (health maintenance organizations) to respond to this challenge, which helped them to share the costs of providing services. I remember clearly in the early 1990s, in the small town of Auburn, California, watching as one MD after another switched from a private practice model to a group practice, or joined a larger organization that provided healthcare. It seemed to happen first with the family practice and general practice providers, then the specialists. Within the larger provider groups or health insurance networks, emphasis was placed on efficiency and frankly, limiting the amount of care provided in order to maximize profit. If you have never seen Michael Moore's film *Sicko* (1), it is a profound insight into this process that seeks to reduce money spent, often to the extremes of causing further disability and even death to people who thought they were covered by their insurance. It gives a very clear picture of the distressing state of medical care at this point in its decline.

In order to be competitive, services over the ensuing years became less focused on the individual and more on the outcome...which might at first sound not so bad, but in fact, the outcome was not only whether the individual (or actually "the diagnosis") was well treated, but whether he or she returned to work. If that person returned to work, the emphasis was on whether their productivity remained the same or worsened/improved.

The providers and companies giving the healthcare knew that if they didn't keep the huge groups of businesses and government payers happy, they would lose business or be forced out of the market. Many insurance companies folded or were bought out, reducing both competition and choice for people like you and me. We talk today of the "Citizens United" decision in the Supreme Court that gave businesses immense power to influence politics and elections, but the same businesses and groups took over your healthcare well before this.

What did all this mean for you, though? You may have had to lose a provider that you loved and trusted for years. He or she may have treated you since you were a child, might have treated your parents or your children. They may have understood you, your family, your business or work, the community, your history, and cared deeply about you. You may have had to switch to a provider who seemed nice, but was rushed, didn't remember you, or treated you like an appointment instead of a person. You may not have been able to see them as much. You started to have to ask permission to see other providers who were specialists, even those that you had seen for years as well.

If you are old enough, do you remember what it was like to see a doctor before this change? This was a typical conversation between someone and their doctor 25 years ago:

Fred: Hi Doctor Forsythe, I'm glad you could get me in today!

Doctor Forsythe: Fred, great to see you again. How's your business going?

Fred: It's doing pretty good, but I couldn't go in today, I have this burning in my stomach.

Doctor Forsythe: Ahhh! Are you eating at that restaurant on the corner again?! (Laughter.)

Doctor Forsythe would then ask questions about Fred's pain...when it started, whether it was there all the time or once in awhile, what set it off or made it better, his diet, his alcohol intake, many other questions, but importantly these questions almost entirely focused on Fred's symptoms and worries **about what he came in for,** and the things that most likely could be occurring. The doctor would jot a few notes, but most of the time would look at Fred and **listen** to him. A much more extensive physical exam was done than usually occurs now, and if Doctor Forsythe was good at what he/she did, would came up with an idea of what could be causing Fred's problem, order tests, then develop a plan that included changes in lifestyle and medications, or more urgent treatment, including surgery if needed or referral to a specialist. Every day Doctor Forsythe would write notes into a paper chart and file them away in the chart room.

Now, it wasn't perfect...doctors didn't have access to all the research quickly, and usually didn't have access to computer programs and the internet that could help them make the diagnosis or give clues to treatments. They used the books in their office, or would call another doctor. They couldn't see all the things that other doctors had done, even if they ordered records and reviewed them. They at times (and still) spoke in terms that make them seem superior or removed, or that were even incomprehensible. They sometimes chose treatments incorrectly. They were definitely human. What they did have was the ability to focus their attention on your problem and your worries and center their help on them with you. They could bring to bear the amazing gifts that people have: their mind, their reasoning, their intuition and wisdom. And probably most importantly, they could form an alliance with you...which research has shown (an annoyingly common phrase, sorry), **is the most important aspect in healing.**

At the point that this transition in the 1990s occurred, however, you could expect exchanges more like the following:

Doctor Forsythe: Hi Frank!

Sam: No my name is Sam...do you remember me??

Doctor Forsythe: (Flustered) Of course! How is your father?

Sam: He died 4 years ago...are you sure you remember me?

Doctor Forsythe: Yes I'm sorry. What can I do for you today?

Sam: You wanted me to come back in two months to check on that new medicine...but I couldn't get in until this month.....

Doctor Forsythe: (recovering) yes, are you having any side effects?

Sam: well, it may be causing trouble with my, you know, in the bed with my wife...

Doctor Forsythe: well, that can be a lot of things...let's try this new medicine to help.

Sam: Well there may be other things going on, too, but...

Doctor Forsythe: well let's try this medicine first, and if it doesn't help, I'll refer you to a therapist... And please make another appointment for two months...

Unfortunately, the amount of time that could be given for each visit grew smaller over the years, and the total number of people that the doctor had responsibility for increased alarmingly. Services were cut, and classes and groups substituted for direct care. I've joked in the past (I have a very dark sense of humor at times) that one day there will be a "Chest Pain Class" to screen people with chest pain, with (hopefully) ambulances nearby.

Emphasis was put on efficiency and speed, and when care faltered, especially in this hyper-competitive environment, more emphasis on the statistics of each provider, hospital, and health plan was made, looking for ways to produce better outcomes with increasing numbers of people per doctor. What was happening was the weakening of the healing relationship, and the growth of statistical analysis was driving competition. It started out about the money, and continues today to be about the money.

The emphasis on statistical analysis and a reasonable desire to coordinate services to provide greater profit for both the insurers and the buyers led in part to the next huge change in healthcare...the computer.

Chapter Two: The Machines and Their Attendants

It has become appallingly obvious that our technology has exceeded our humanity.

Albert Einstein

If you've ever seen the movie "Moneyball" (2), you know it is the remarkable story of the Oakland A's and their revolution in outcomes and success driven by a shift to the statistical analysis of players abilities and outcomes, which decreased the focus on star players and increased the focus on teamwork, resulting in an improvement in their scoring. It worked, because while fans are connected to the individual players, they are also were proud to be connected to a team. If you could more consistently produce more runs, you could consistently produce more wins. Oakland was so successful, their methods were adopted by other teams who, having more money, eventually eclipsed the A's success.

This approach was increasingly applied to medical care, and in focusing on improving outcomes; it was used also to improve the competitive edge for groups of providers and healthcare systems, resulting in hopeful increased profits and survival of the healthcare organization. It is important to state that an "outcome" is a piece of data, and not you! So if your survival, for example, from cancer extended another 6 months or a year, that's an improved outcome, even if it was miserable for you.

The problem is that in healthcare (versus a ball club), while there is an effect of being seen at or connected to an organization that consistently has a great reputation, e.g. Stanford Medical Center, the connection and alliance with the provider is even more powerful and vital to healing in healthcare than fans' adoration of a star baseball hitter or pitcher.

Our computers are marvelous at this statistical analysis, and can not only look at statistics on an individual doctor's care, but also compare these to multiple other providers, multiple other patients/clients, and contrast this with many research studies to provide "recommendations" about what should be done in your specific instance.

On the surface of it, it would appear to be a wonderful improvement in caring for you. How can you fully argue with better outcomes and improved coordination of care?? Unfortunately, at least two things went very wrong in the process.

First, for the computer and the people looking at its output to know what the doctor is doing, the doctor has to type information into the computer, so it can monitor what is happening. This is not just what the doctor thinks is going on and what he or she is planning on doing to treat your problem, **but all the steps leading up to it.**

For example, in his or her approach to a patient, after his or her greetings and the personal exchanges of meeting (see chapter one), the doctor asks questions about the problem bringing you in. You're also asked questions that may or may not relate to the problem (more about this later). Your blood pressure is taken, your weight, and sometimes other measurements, all entered into the computer. Finally, the doctor examines you. Then, tests are reviewed and other tests are often ordered. An assessment of the problem is made, a plan of treatment is developed, and referrals to other specialists, if needed, are arranged. Medicines are often prescribed. A follow up visit is planned.

In the past, much of this was written by hand, often in a very abbreviated form, onto paper. Now however, in addition to the all the activities above, the doctor types all of this into the record. Remember, the time the doctor is given with you is now limited due to efforts to be more efficient and "productive," ignoring that there is that very thorny problem of the doctor taking some time to reflect on what is happening with you.

In the rush to see more and more people, with increasing requirements to enter all the aspects of the visit into the machine, there is less and less time for the doctor to 1. Listen to you, 2. Connect with you as a person and 3. Use his or her intuition, knowledge and experience to arrive at an understanding of what the problem is and how to treat it.

You can begin to see what, about 10 years ago, led to an ever increasing distance between you and the doctor. These human doctors, no better or worse than you, were starting to lose the time to listen to you, to think about you, to use their wisdom and alliance with you. To provide the data needed to their computer, they had to develop an increasingly intimate relationship with their machines, and increasingly had to rely on them (and fear the consequences of not giving them the data they required, much like the hungry plant Audrey II in Little Shop of Horrors).

The second problem was that the data was increasingly analyzed. The computers for their part, provided information to their analysts. While this certainly can provide help (e.g. outright mistakes, "Why are you using birth control pills to treat a common cold?!"), it more often led to more requests and requirements for even more information. So it wasn't enough to see if what your doctor did was working, but the analysis led to focusing on all the steps in between...including what questions you've been asked, what kind of exam was done, which tests were ordered, what kind what medicines you've been prescribed, and so on. With outcomes **and** money being the bottom line, all of these were subject to scrutiny and potential analysis and criticism, so even if you are happy with your care, even if you feel an alliance with your doctor, even if you are feeling better, it's not enough. The statistics are paramount. The people who pay for your care (assuming it's not you), want more done with less money, which again means less time. The costs of tests, medicines, treatments, time off for you, number of visits needed, consultations, specialist referrals, all are weighed and assessed.

Again, while some of this helps you at times, the end result on the doctor is increasing pressure to document...not just to avoid lawsuits anymore, but to avoid the pressures from the analysis and analysts to document and alter care, and avoid potentially the risk of losing their jobs or, if still in private practice, watch their income decline due to being unable to implement all the analysts' requirements.

While it would be nice to opt out of this computerized system, both for you and your provider, it's no longer possible in most settings to abandon the computers, their analysts and these demands, because if providers fail to have or develop an Electronic Health Record system (EHR) and follow all of the guidelines, they will face increasing monetary penalties.

The final result of this stage was that more and more, doctors and other providers have become simply attendants entering data into the machines, for analysis by someone who has very little or no understanding of what happened at your visit. That person is probably very much more interested in the data he or she is analyzing and whether it will show results that are favorable to the healthcare initiatives they've proposed.

The computers assessing you and your doctor can only analyze what the analysts have programmed into it...it is not really taking in all the unique and important information that exists in that office, but samples of information that can never form a whole view of what is really important in your care.

So you were already seeing someone who was rushed in the first place, often knew or remembered you less, and now that provider has to satisfy an increasing number of analysts of data who have the power to make life extremely hard for the provider.

Now you could expect conversations like this:

Doctor Forsythe: So nice to see you again Ms. Pate. What brings you in today?

Sarah: I've had this weird pain in my foot for about 4 weeks...it's burning and seems to be getting worse, off and on...and I....

Doctor Forsythe: (typing into his computer) have you ever had a similar pain? When? What makes it worse? What makes it better? Do you have a family history of weird pains in the foot? What were you doing when it first started hurting? Is it worse in the morning... Hold on one second...OK, is it worse in the morning or at night, does it...

Fred: Doctor, I really need you to look at my foot!

Doctor Forsythe: just a couple more things I have to fill in...

Fred: Doctor, I know you're rushed, but could you look at me for a moment...you're typing into your computer and I really need to talk to you....

Had this been the final change to care, again starting about 10 years ago, doctors might have gradually adapted, and you might be getting a little of the personal, caring connection you had in the 80s...but as we seem to create what we envision, both in our hopes and fears (look at the dystopian movies that are so popular), the analysts and their machines became even more powerful.

Chapter Three: Who Are the Analysts?

There is nothing more ominous than a meeting room full of people, all wanting to get ahead, with "wonderful" ideas.
Paul Jurkowski

It is easy enough to blame the doctor who provides care. You may have felt completely disregarded, unheard, just another appointment in their schedule, meaning nothing to them. They may have even been outright disrespectful and condescending to you. You think, "They make plenty of money, they have privilege, they are out of touch." Sometimes, you are very right. I have certainly met other doctors who seem by their very nature NOT to like people...who are condescending and judgmental--judging clients for a background of drug use, or tattoos, or lifestyle choices. I have met doctors who judged people for their weight, or for their children's weight...one that even felt that parents of overweight children should be turned into a social service agency for child abuse. Doctors like this have little understanding of life; for example, how hard it is to feed children on a minimum wage (or less) with healthy food.

Most of the time, however, you'll be wrong. I'll describe in the next chapter what is happening to doctors that leave them distant and seemingly uncaring. In most cases doctors go into to medicine not for the lure of prestige and money, but much more for their caring nature, their love of science, and the amazing adventure of figuring out how things happen to you and how you can be helped. Some do outside work with charity organizations in addition to what they do at work and time spent with their family. They are often lovely people at heart.

If you don't blame the provider, you can then blame the organization they work for: "XYZ Healthcare only thinks about profits, they don't care about their patients/clients." You'll be right some of the time, but again, I think you're missing the bigger picture. Healthcare has been under siege for many years. It's not just company XYZ. Many companies have gone out of business after losing the battle, and those that are left, whether they admit it or not, are scared...more scared than a roomful of stock traders, even if they're doing well.

In my mind, you'd be closer to the truth if you look at where the money is, and our failure (all of our failures) to guarantee healthcare for everyone, but that still is not the full truth. Remember, increasing desire for money for healthcare and concern for profits started this mess, worsened it when companies and groups got angry about costs and forced more and more services for less, and worsened still more when we became hungry for more data to make healthcare more "efficient" (more for less). Healthcare companies certainly could have taken a higher road and tried more earnestly to limit premium increases, but their fear of becoming insolvent and that universal human desire for safety (no matter the cost in public perception of that organization) pushes increases in fees.

Perhaps the greatest problem, which truly had been there before, but only as a seedling, threatens to destroy what little is left in your relationship with your provider...the explosion of analysis, and the resulting regulations based on that analysis.

While organizations and providers struggled to deal with their machines, increasingly, more and more regulations have been written in stone about what is or isn't necessary in the computer documentation and what is or isn't required in the doctors responses and the outcomes. Healthcare organizations cannot survive if they don't comply with these regulations...they can lose huge sums of money. Individual providers can opt out of this for now, but the pressure on them builds yearly.

Remember we talked about the doctor's focus on your problem back in the 80s (and before) and the questions asked that focused on **your** difficulty? Now the analysts have come up with an ever-widening set of required questions and interventions to be asked or suggested by your provider. Each of these usually is based on research, good intentions, desire to improve healthcare, and probably most importantly, to look good in the analyst's meetings...brilliant, cutting edge, even witty! (OK, I'm joking, but only in part.) So you can't really argue with the idea that at your visit your doctor should ask you about:

Alcohol use, drug use, cigarette or tobacco use, presence of second hand smoke in your environment, domestic violence, diet and exercise (how much, how often), whether or not you've completed your routine vaccinations or screening exams,

whether you're sexually active, using safe sex practices, what

medicines you're taking and if you miss any, what over the

counter or herbal medicines you're taking, have you been injured

by a third party, have you traveled and been exposed to serious

illnesses and so on. (Yes, there are more, and unless meetings

become illegal, there will be even more.) You might be horrified

that I even suggest that these aren't important, but I'm not

suggesting that at all. Think about it--each of these can be vital,

but now you have:

(From Chapter One):

Doctor Forsythe would then ask questions about Fred's

pain...when it started, whether it was there all the time or

once in awhile, what set it off or made it better, his diet, his

alcohol intake, many other questions, but importantly

almost entirely focused on Fred's symptoms and worries

about what he came in for, and the things that most likely could be occurring. If Doctor Forsythe was good at what he did, he came up with an idea of what could be causing Fred's problem, then ordered tests. He would come up with a plan that included changes in lifestyle and medications, or more urgent treatment, including surgery if needed or seeing a specialist. Every day Doctor Forsythe would write his notes into a paper chart and file them away in the chart room.

(From Chapter Two):

In the past, much of this was written by hand, often in a very abbreviated form, onto paper. Now, in addition to the all the activities above, the doctor types all of this into the record. Oh, and let's not forget that the time the doctor is given with you is now limited due to efforts to be more efficient and "productive" ignoring that very thorny problem of the doctor taking some time to reflect on what is happening with you!

In the rush to see more and more people, with increasing requirements to enter all the aspects of the visit into the machine, there is less and less time for the doctor to 1. Listen to you, 2. Connect with you as a person and 3. Use his or her ability, intuition and knowledge.

And now:

Alcohol use, drug use, cigarette or tobacco use, presence of second hand smoke in your environment, domestic violence, diet and exercise (how much, how often), whether or not you've completed your routine vaccinations or screening exams, whether you're sexually active, using safe sex practices, what medicines you're taking and if you miss any, what over the counter or herbal medicines you're taking,

have you been injured by a third party, have you traveled and been exposed to serious illnesses and so on...

Sometimes people are asked these same questions repeatedly, even when they are seeing providers on a regular basis for a chronic problem throughout the year.

Now, if you're lucky, very lucky, your doctor may have 30 minutes to do this, but much more likely, there will be about 15 minutes to do all of this. Today much of the time that could be used to talk with you and ask you questions that are primarily focused on your problem is used for asking questions that fulfill regulatory requirements for documentation, OFTEN AT EVERY VISIT. Usually, you will get very little of those 15 minutes for your concerns.

Functioning in this environment for a provider becomes something like it must be at a major disaster, e.g. a plane crash.

You have to make a rapid assessment, and your determination will be based on recognizing patterns of illness that are common. Once that determination is made, the doctor proceeds, and can be very dismissive of any objections or additional information you try to bring up. He or she is headed down their path, and doesn't want to rethink the decision with so little time left. You have been cubby holed, and often there you stay.

After you leave, the regulatory influences don't end there, and to understand more, we need to look at some of the governmental agencies that are involved.

If you look at a **partial** list of agencies involved in oversight of healthcare you'll be amazed. In a recent article (in an excellent medical education website, Medscape), called Building Healthcare Delivery Around Quality: Implementing the National Quality Strategy (3), more than 40 agencies were identified in promoting the "National Quality Strategy".

The Centers for Medicare and Medicaid Services (CMS), and the Office of the National Coordinator for Health Information Technology (ONC), while not the only groups involved in analysis and regulation of healthcare, are two of the most powerful influences on medical care today. The article goes on to state:

"There are currently more than 40 programs, each designed to address one or more priorities, under the stewardship of multiple federal agencies, representing private-sector, federal, state, and local efforts."

If you want some eye-opening reading plow through this article--it's mind numbing, and while each of these programs almost certainly have caring and committed people in them, remember, they have meetings, and come up with recommendations, which often then get passed on to CMS (the Centers for Medicaid and Medicare Services), which then as the administering agency, can pass on as "guidelines"/regulations to healthcare providers.

What comes out of CMS? They administer Medicaid and Medicare, both absolutely vital programs. **Their recommendations are often put in place for all patients/clients, whether they are covered under Medicare/Medicaid or not.** Unfortunately, while their intent (and ONC's) may be good, their output is this: more requirements.

A large part of these regulations, as an example, are the "Meaningful Use" requirements. These have been brought out in stages, beginning in 2010. Read the following only if you want to get a full sense of the enormity of the regulations health care providers face...or you can skip ahead if you'd like.

As of 2010, stage one consisted, according to the CMS website (4) of:

Meaningful Use Core Objectives

Eligible Professionals--15 Core Objectives

1. Computerized Provider Order Entry (CPOE)

2. E-Prescribing (eRx)

3. Report ambulatory clinical quality measures to CMS/States

4. Implement one clinical decision support rule

5. Provide patients with an electronic copy of their health information, upon request

6. Provide clinical summaries for patients for each office visit

7. Drug-drug and drug-allergy interaction checks

8. Record demographics

9. Maintain an up-to-date problem list of current and active diagnoses

10. Maintain active medication list

11. Maintain active medication allergy list

12. Record and chart changes in vital signs

13. Record smoking status for patients 13 years or older

14. Capability to exchange key clinical information among providers of care and patient-authorized entities electronically

15. Protect electronic health information

2. Menu objectives-may defer 5 out of 10

Eligible Professionals--10 Menu Objectives

1. Drug-formulary checks

2. Incorporate clinical lab test results as structured data

3. Generate lists of patients by specific conditions

4. Send reminders to patients per patient preference for preventive/follow up care

5. Provide patients with timely electronic access to their health information

6. Use certified EHR technology to identify patient-specific education resources and provide to patient, if appropriate

7. Medication reconciliation

8. Summary of care record for each transition of care/referrals

9. Capability to submit electronic data to immunization registries/systems*

10. Capability to provide electronic syndromic surveillance data to public health agencies*

* At least 1 public health objective must be selected

3. MU: Clinical Quality Measures

Clinical Quality Measures (CQM) Core CQM

Eligible Professionals must complete 3 of the following:

Hypertension – Blood Pressure Measurement Preventive

Care and Screening Measure Pair Tobacco Use Assessment

Tobacco Cessation Intervention

Adult Weight Screening and Follow up

Weight Assessment and Counseling for Children and Adolescents

Preventive Care and Screening

Influenza Immunization for Patients > 50 Years old

Childhood Immunization Status

Additional Set CQM--EPs must complete 3 of 38

1. Diabetes: Hemoglobin A1c Poor Control

2. Diabetes: Low Density Lipoprotein (LDL) Management and Control

3. Diabetes: Blood Pressure Management

4. Heart Failure (HF): Angiotensin-Converting Enzyme (ACE) Inhibitor or Angiotensin Receptor Blocker (ARB) Therapy for Left Ventricular Systolic Dysfunction (LVSD)

5. Coronary Artery Disease (CAD): Beta-Blocker Therapy for CAD Patients with Prior Myocardial Infarction (MI)

6. Pneumonia Vaccination Status for Older Adults

7. Breast Cancer Screening

8. Colorectal Cancer Screening

9. Coronary Artery Disease (CAD): Oral Antiplatelet Therapy Prescribed for Patients with CAD

10. Heart Failure (HF): Beta-Blocker Therapy for Left Ventricular Systolic Dysfunction (LVSD)

11. Anti-depressant medication management: (a) Effective Acute Phase Treatment, (b) Effective Continuation Phase Treatment

12. **Primary Open Angle Glaucoma (POAG): Optic Nerve Evaluation**

Diabetic Retinopathy: Documentation of Presence or Absence of Macular Edema and Level of Severity of Retinopathy

13. **Diabetic Retinopathy: Communication with the Physician Managing Ongoing Diabetes Care**

15. **Asthma Pharmacologic Therapy**

16. **Asthma Assessment**

17. **Appropriate Testing for Children with Pharyngitis 18. Oncology Breast Cancer: Hormonal Therapy for Stage IC-IIIC Estrogen Receptor/Progesterone Receptor (ER/ PR) Positive Breast Cancer**

19. **Oncology Colon Cancer: Chemotherapy for Stage III Colon Cancer Patients**

20. Prostate Cancer: Avoidance of Overuse of Bone Scan for Staging Low Risk Prostate Cancer Patients

21. Smoking and Tobacco Use Cessation, Medical Assistance: a) Advising Smokers and Tobacco Users to Quit, b) Discussing Smoking and Tobacco Use Cessation Medications, c) Discussing Smoking and Tobacco Use Cessation Strategies

22. Diabetes: Eye Exam

23. Diabetes: Urine Screening

24. Diabetes: Foot Exam

25. Coronary Artery Disease (CAD): Drug Therapy for Lowering LDL-Cholesterol

26. Heart Failure (HF): Warfarin Therapy Patients with Atrial Fibrillation

27. Ischemic Vascular Disease (IVD): Blood Pressure Management

28. **Ischemic Vascular Disease (IVD): Use of Aspirin or Another Antithrombotic**

29. **Initiation and Engagement of Alcohol and Other Drug Dependence Treatment: a) Initiation, b)Engagement**

30. **Prenatal Care: Screening for Human Immunodeficiency Virus (HIV)**

31. **Prenatal Care: Anti-D Immune Globulin**

32. **Controlling High Blood Pressure**

33. **Cervical Cancer Screening**

34. **Chlamydia Screening for Women**

35. **Use of Appropriate Medications for Asthma**

36. **Low Back Pain: Use of Imaging Studies**

37. **Ischemic Vascular Disease (IVD): Complete Lipid Panel and LDL Control**

38. **Diabetes: Hemoglobin A1c Control (<8.0%)**

The amazing thing is that this was only Stage 1---in 2014, Stage 2 began its "roll-out." This established an **additional 42** objectives (requirements) that your doctor will have to follow, very similar to the types listed above, but in fact even more complex. Some of these multiple new recommendations also rely on you to provide follow up documentation to your doctor, but even if you don't, you won't be penalized, the provider will. I won't list the new set...you get the idea.

What is important to realize here is that the regulators and analysts are attempting to create a regulatory, electronic brain with its own decision pathways that substitute for the training and expertise of the doctor, in essence supplanting his or her decision making, (which should depend heavily on your circumstances). There is every indication that they will continue:

they have planned a Stage 3, coming out perhaps in 2018, and will likely continue on with further stages.

All of this potentially severely impacts the meeting you have with your provider, and while its intentions are good, in practice what happens is that the provider is under more pressure to satisfy these requirements in his interactions with you, whether face to face, or increasingly, by electronic communications, e.g. e mails.

This brings up a final point for this chapter: 25 years ago, the doctor made some phone calls during and at the end of their day, reviewed tests, and finished up their notes, and went home. Increasingly now, the doctor spends more and more time communicating with clients and professionals electronically, despite often having a fully scheduled day of face-to-face visits. This often means that work will be done at home as well. Remember, the number of clients has dramatically increased, so the number of interactions a provider has with clients that are not face to face has also increased dramatically. The provider may not remember you, because you haven't been able to see them for several months. You may have seen several other providers in the meantime, all of them new to you. Often if you can't get in to see your provider, even with problems ranging from minor to very serious, you are now e mailing or leaving voice mails, so the "after hours" or "in between appointments" work is increasingly more time consuming and can consist of problems that are very serious in nature. Often the provider, who certainly knows you better than an emergency room provider, will have to refer you to the ER out of fear of what will happen to you overnight (if you're lucky enough to get an appointment the next day), or until you're seen several days later.

In the movie *Gallipoli* (4), depicting the assault on the Ottoman Empire during World War One, there is a tragic scene showing waves of Allied infantry trying to capture Turkish positions on the "V" beach. The Turks had mounted machine guns pointed at the beachhead, and as each wave came off the boats and across the beach, they were gunned down by the hundreds. The generals communicated through wired telegraph to the troop commanders. The generals were off shore in ships, and could not see the carnage happening in the assault. They continued to order assault after assault, blind to the realities and historic tragedy they were causing.

Much like those generals, without a knowledge of what is actually happening in health care...current knowledge and direct experience of what is happening in the office, the analysts have, with all good intentions, helped destroy the healing relationship.

Sitting in meetings, probably perusing algorithms and statistics and flow charts, the blows are struck again and again.

We now increasingly find even less understanding of your desires and needs:

Doctor Forsythe: I see you're in for a skin problem.... can I ask you a few questions first?

Fred: Well, sure, but...

Doctor Forsythe: (typing) I see that you checked yes on your form that you use alcohol and tobacco...also the computer tells me that you are late for your flu shot, and you need a sigmoidoscopy, and...

Fred: Yes, but

Doctor Forsythe: (typing, staring intently at the computer, very stressed and short with Fred) just a moment, let's get this entered and we'll talk more about your face. By the way, is there any violence at home? Are you using any drugs besides alcohol? Have you been traveling outside the country?

Fred: Doc....

Doctor Forsyth: Look, I just have a few questions more...

Fred: **Look at my face!**

Doctor Forsythe: oh, that looks like eczema...here is a prescription for a cream and here is a summary of our visit today...make an appointment with the receptionist for a follow up visit in 6 weeks (typing). I'll send you an e-mail with all my contact numbers...(leaves exam room, off to the next computer interaction).

Fred: but you didn't really examine me...

This client is feeling increasingly lost. In chapter four, we'll look at what is happening to your provider.

Chapter Four: The Spirit of Caring Under Assault

Burnout is nature's way of telling you, you've been going through the motions, your soul has departed; you're a zombie, a member of the walking dead, a sleepwalker. False optimism is like administrating stimulants to an exhausted nervous system.

Sam Keen, *Fire in the Belly: On Being a Man*

The rate of successful suicide in physicians is somewhere around double that of our general population. The rates of mental disorders in physicians are increasing as well. About 400 physicians take their life yearly in the U.S., usually by firearms or overdose. As doctors understand how the body works, their completion rate of suicide attempts is higher than with most people. They are often diagnosed with depression or substance use, but are less willing to seek help for it, as the stigma we still give to these problems can potentially affect their career.

I was a psychiatrist for most of my years in practice, and I've noticed that there can be a final reckoning in some peoples' minds when someone commits suicide, once they have received a "diagnosis." "Poor Doc, he/she had problems with depression." If we look at depression as an illness, dependent more on genetics than stress, it's easier to write off what happens as a particular vulnerability, a "weakness" (though in truth, we all have vulnerabilities). However, in my mind, depression is more of an injury, and stress plays a huge role in that injury. Given enough stress, perhaps everyone can become depressed.

Scientists conducted a horrifying experiment many years ago that resulted in a concept called "learned helplessness." They essentially locked dogs in cages and shocked them repeatedly to see what would happen. The dogs were angry and scared and fought back at first, but then when they couldn't stop the repeated shocks, they withdrew, shook, their appetite and sleep were poor, they gave up, all mimicking human depression.

Under enough prolonged stress, I think anyone can come to this point, doctors included. It arises from a set of conditions in which the suffering increases, and the ability to take action to ease the suffering decreases. Some doctors turn to drugs and alcohol to ease the stress, and then these become new problems in and of themselves, again hidden from other doctors and supervisors to avoid the stigma and loss of job/livelihood.

You probably won't have a provider who takes his or her own life, but you are much more likely to experience "burn out" in your provider. What this might feel like to you may be leaving the office thinking that your worries or feelings are not important to the provider, or feeling you were the target of sarcasm or outright anger during the visit. At a minimum, the doctor seemed distracted or distant.

What is "burn out" exactly? In an article by Carol Peckham, a Medscape contributor, titled "Physician Burnout: It Just Keeps Getting Worse" in January of 2015 (6), it is described as "...loss of enthusiasm for work, feelings of cynicism, and a low sense of personal accomplishment..." Additionally there is a numbing of sensitivity to clients. In Medscape reports including the above citation, this burnout has increased from about 9% in 2010, to just under 40% in 2013, to 46% on average currently, for physicians as a whole. The rate is actually higher in primary care doctors and other front line specialties.

This numbing and cynicism worsens your alliance, sometimes even kills it; it may even worsen your care, because as a doctor becomes numb to what you are telling him, (and more focused on inputting data to satisfy the regulators), his or her decisions have to be based less on your input. Also, I suspect that as the numbing increases decision making itself becomes impaired, even with all the information available. The doctor's mind is distracted, operating poorly, attempting to multitask to the point that potentially nothing is done well.

Yet how can a doctor not feel less enthusiasm when his assessment and actions are increasingly picked for him, his time for assessment limited? This would of course lead to a low sense of personal accomplishment. And in the end, given that he or she can be left feeling like an extension of the regulations and the computer and its analysts, why wouldn't they feel cynical?

There is an aspect of the provider's experience in some that the burnout scenario doesn't capture however, and that is the increasing fear and anxiety in doctors. This is not something talked about much, but it can be terrifying to come in to work with huge caseloads, especially when it becomes easier to make mistakes with increasingly less time for more and more decisions. And if there have been bad outcomes (patients harmed or who have died), the fear becomes much worse. In my mind this is much worse than the fear of malpractice that doctors had in the past (which also still exists as well and overlaps this fear).

Burnout can potentially result in serious mistakes, very tragic for you, and additionally tragic because your provider was probably once a very bright, caring person.

The rate of doctors leaving practice and pursuing non-clinical jobs is increasing. Physicians like me who had retirement available may take it sooner rather than later. The impact on medical care, **your care,** can be devastating.

This book, though, is not written to sing a funeral dirge for the old doctor-client relationship, but to help you understand what is going on so that you can take steps to protect yourself, and also so that you can understand that **none of this is about you personally.** You are struggling to be heard and cared for in a system that is breaking. At times providers will give you the impression that this is your problem and that you're being unreasonable, that you're asking for too much. While you do need to make healthy choices for your life, and that responsibility lies solely with you, the responses you get from a failing system are not at all your fault.

Chapter Five: It's Not Just The Doctors

Great work is not ordinarily done in busyness.

Elizabeth Skoglund, author and psychotherapist

I recently went with a friend to an appointment in a cardiology department at a large hospital. I sat with her in the waiting room--she was waiting to be fitted with a Holter monitor, a device that records your heart rhythm over 24 hours to see whether you have problems with your rhythm that could be serious.

We arrived early, and as we waited, there was a family, seemingly a father and mother and their son. The father was in a wheelchair. Neither parent spoke English, and the son was translating for them. He was trying very hard to get a staff member to help him understand how he could get follow up for his parents. She couldn't tell him the correct number, but she said, half-heartedly, that they could try another number and they might get connected to the right number through whoever answered that line. When the son protested, the woman told him that was all she could do. The staff never smiled, and clearly just wanted to get out of the waiting room. The son and his parents left.

My friend went in for her appointment. The woman who came out for her looked exhausted and irritated. My friend told me that when she put the electrodes on for the device, she scraped her skin until it was very abraded and painful. When she got home, she found parts of the taping that were supposed to be removed and weren't. I asked her if they gave her a log when I was driving her home, and she said, "No, she just put these on and left." (You're supposed to keep a log of how you feel when hooked up to the device, so that if you feel weak or dizzy or feel sensations in your chest, they can check to see if this is connected to the rhythm of your heart.) Later, she found the log in a bag that the staff had handed her without a word. My friend is very reliable and not prone to drama or exaggeration. It was disheartening to see her and the family in the waiting room treated this way.

Coincidence? Probably not. The stresses on doctors also are exerted on their staff. Often staff bears most of the criticism from clients, as many people are afraid to assert themselves with the doctor. It can be frightening to be assertive or get angry with someone who makes decisions that affect your life, and it can be easier to try and blame staff for problems in a department.

You have probably read about strikes by staff, nurses, therapists, clerical workers, etc. Doctors in most systems are not unionized and so won't strike, but this is not an indication that they are happier with their jobs.

The systems in healthcare are trying to juggle responsibilities to clients, the buyer groups and government, and all of their employees can suffer in the process.

For you, you need to understand that no one has a right to treat you this way, and that you deserve better, humane treatment. On a financial level, on average, you or the company you work for is paying about 12,000 dollars yearly for your care. Is this what you'd expect for that much money?

Even if burned out staff imply that you are the problem, **this is not about you.** If you're rude, fine, you can be blamed for your actions, but much of the time it is the exhaustion, fear, or anger **in the staff** that you're experiencing. They can be terrified of losing their job, feeling pressured, and feeling trapped, and when people feel trapped, at least at first, they can get defensive and fight back. Later, the numbing process begins, which is what I think was happening in the two staff that saw my friend and that family.

Chapter Six: Taking Your Care Back

Get up, stand up, Stand up for your rights. Get up, stand up, don't give up the fight.

Bob Marley

When you walk into a provider's office, you are asking for help, compassion, expertise. It is **your** health, not your doctors. It is **your** health, not the organization he or she works for. It is **your** health, not the government's. It is your time, your health, and the doctor is supposed to be there for you. If all these changes have happened in healthcare, is it hopeless?

To give you an idea of what can happen in a doctor's office today that is NOT in your best interest, I'll illustrate by describing a visit related to me by a friend (not one of my own clients). This visit was not as serious as some, but illustrates perfectly the potential for problems. Contrast this to the visit described in Chapter One as you read:

An 18-year-old girl came to an appointment with her MD. Her main complaint was a sore throat and fatigue that had lasted for weeks. She was dating, but not steady with anyone.

During the course of the visit, her doctor asked her rightfully about sexual activity, but seemed to focus as well on multiple other screening questions that involved required health screens under the new guidelines. In the 15 minute visit the young woman had little or no time to describe what has happened to her over the last several weeks, but instead found out that she needed a gynecological visit, should get two vaccines she was due for, including a flu vaccine (feeling as badly as she did), after the visit. Smoking, drug use, alcohol use, presence of violence in the home, multiple other areas that had only peripheral meaning to her problem were assessed. She did have a throat culture done, but no blood tests.

Many parents, perhaps especially mothers, and most doctors are screaming right now: "She probably has Mono"! That idea was not discussed, by all appearances not considered, and not tested for at this visit. The difficulty of not finding infectious mononucleosis at a doctors visit is that there are occasional complications including potentially serious rupture of an internal organ (the spleen), and a higher risk for a secondary infections.

She certainly had all the regulatory measures checked off. I suspect the MD, if given the time to just sit for a few minutes and focus on her problem and let his marvelous mind with all of its wisdom **reflect** on what was going on, he might have thought about it, discussed it with her, ordered a simple blood test to screen for it, and cautioned her against physical contact sports to avoid the potential for a ruptured spleen. She survived this episode, little thanks to the MD or all the wonderful ideas regulators have come up with in all those important meetings. The doctor simply didn't have enough time to bring his focus to her problem. He was focused on fulfilling obligations to an ever-increasing set of rules and requirements with less time, and with more patients waiting in the waiting room and attempting to communicate with him electronically and by phone. Had she had a bad result, **he** would have been the focus of any actions, lawsuits or otherwise, not the system of healthcare in this country. The system will assign blame to the provider, despite creating conditions that undermine that provider's ability to use his or her training and intuition. From our point of view, of course it will be clear that he indeed made the mistake that caused harm. However if that same provider were trying to care for the injured in a train wreck, we would give him or her more latitude. What can't be seen by the computer analysts (and is often hidden from you), is that this is exactly what the provider is in the midst of: a train wreck.

Now, I want to stop here and talk about politics and healthcare. Some could use what I'm saying to further their fight against governmental control of healthcare: "You see, the government screwed it up again! We need to let our free enterprise system handle healthcare! I knew Obamacare was _____" (Fill in communist, socialist, a terrible idea, government overreach, etc.)

Nothing could be further from the truth. For profit healthcare and the market system had many, many years to get it right, and didn't. At the time that the Affordable Care Act or "Obamacare" went into effect, 45 million people had no healthcare, and every year about one of every 1000 of them died (about 45,000). In one study, if you received urgent care for multiple trauma from, for example, a car accident, and weren't insured, you were 33% more likely to die than someone with insurance.

Now at least as I am writing this there are 17 million more people with coverage. That may be 17,000 more people who live this year, and 17 million adults and children who don't have to live in fear of needing care and not having anywhere to turn. What we really need urgently is **everyone** covered, through a Medicare plan for each person in our country. If you take a Darwinian "survival of the fittest" stance on this, and feel that healthcare is a privilege, not a right, I will suggest that survival of the fittest species as an idea is brilliant, but it is incomplete. It is NOT just survival of the fittest species, but survival of the fittest **system**...meaning that a system that is complex and **interdependent** will survive and be the most resilient, or to put it another way, we all get there together. This country will be at its greatest if it works together and looks out for all of its citizens.

Others might accuse me of being a Libertarian, because I want less regulation. Again, not true. I do agree that our government regulates too much. In a world where people can be choked to death for reselling cigarettes, and little children get lemonade stands shut down for not having a permit, and healthcare is so regulated that the provider no longer has time to listen, and many other examples, the government has gone too far. Government, however, does need to keep us safe, with police, fire departments, care for the elderly and disabled, education, armed forces, and healthcare. The problem with the current out of touch regulators is that they are not only asking that treatment and outcomes be appropriate for each problem (fair enough since they are giving providers "their" (our) money), they are also (virtually) coming in to the doctor's office and telling him or her how to make assessments and decisions, how to communicate with patients, how to follow up, what to write, how to think, and that if he or she doesn't focus on **their** demands and needs, the provider can find themselves in increasing trouble.

The fact is, understanding how to assess and treat a client was what medical school or graduate school and internship/residency were for.

This is like a grandparent who gives you a box of Legos for your birthday, and then tells you what you have to build, how to build it, how many you need to build, what colors and sizes to use, and demands that you send them daily reports with photos, and also requires that your friends report back to them on your projects. If you don't do all these things, no more Legos for you.

So what do we do to fix this?

There are doctors who are opting out of this crazy system, refusing to follow the guidelines, or even refusing to take Medicare and Medicaid, but it is a relatively small movement, and where does that leave us if we need to provide services to those who can't afford it? Government (and we) will still need to pay one day for healthcare, just like all other developed countries.

There are providers within the system who are daily carving out the time to listen to their clients and really come to an understanding of what is happening with them. They are a true gift, and they are courageous, but remember, it is usually at the expense of very long hours for them and sometimes longer waits for you. This usually can't be sustained for a long period of time, and more importantly, the regulatory requirements for the provider continue to grow, so eventually even the best providers will reach their limit. They need their jobs and income, but are getting exhausted, and are often thinking about leaving.

If you expect businesses and other groups to become suddenly more generous with their money and pay for more care for everyone, so that there will be more time for you to see your provider, it's more likely the sun will change course.

If you expect healthcare companies to draw the line against all the new demands on doctors, think again...remember, they are dependent on reimbursement from governmental agencies and have to toe the line. They still remember the bloodbath of the 90s when multiple healthcare companies were driven out of business.

Finally, if you expect the regulators and analysts, all those people in meetings, in CMS, ONC, and in multiple other groups in both the public and private sectors to decide that they really have made too many recommendations, I can't imagine they will, **unless they have to.** They have occasionally relaxed their timelines and requirements a bit, but coming up with ideas and new rules is in their DNA. The truth is that **unchecked**, they will continue to develop more requirements and further weaken and destroy your relationship with your provider.

I think medical care is improved in some ways by technology, but its human aspect is becoming a hollow shell, and again, this is what does most of the healing, not the regulations or the technology. So how do we push back against these pressures?

The only real way to get your healthcare back is for you to do it at each and every appointment.

I will never forget a client who walked into my office and said "I smoke and I drink, that's who I am, so let's get that out of the way," with a big smile on his face. He was there to discuss a problem, and wasn't willing to change...I still gently suggested he might cut down a bit later in the session, but what I did in that visit and to the best of my ability in all visits, was to make the visit about his needs and worries, and do my best to use my understanding and knowledge to help him. I sat and listened for a long time, asking questions at times, but the questions focused on **his** fears and **his** dilemma, not all the outside analysts' concerns and requirements.

You might meet someone who practices that way, but I came to a point that I couldn't, and so are other MDs. So I have a simple suggestion...if you want to be heard and you want to be able to trust your provider, you **must speak from your heart** and talk about your needs. It doesn't have to be a confrontation...you don't have to attack the doctor or their system or the government or anything else. Let's look at some examples:

Doctor A: I see that you told my assistant that you smoke...and also that you have two glasses of wine a night...do you mind if we talk about this a bit?

You: **maybe in the future**, but **today I only want to talk about** how badly my big toe is hurting...OR

You: **no, I'm not willing to change that for now**...and I'm not here to talk about my exercise, diet, or anything else but my big toe.

Doctor A: but you must understand Ms. B, that your lifestyle can negatively impact all areas of your health...

You: **and I understand you're under pressure to ask me a lot of questions, but I would really like you to stop typing and look at me**..I'm really worried about my big toe...it's turning black and I'm afraid I'm going to lose it.

Doctor A: that's fine but we really must cover those areas...

You: **so let's schedule another visit in the future** and I'll answer all your questions then, but I see now that my toe just fell off on your floor.

Had the doctor focused on your problem and stayed focused on it and you for much of the session you would have an alliance.. You might not have saved your toe, but you now have started to develop a trusting relationship with your provider...and as healthcare **devolves**, you will need to be the one to speak your mind... Also, let's say that your smoking was part of the problem...your circulation to your poor toe was not great because of it. If you felt supported and listened to, you might even be willing to think about quitting one day, but the **trust has to be there first.**

If your doctor is burned out, dismissive, focused on his or her requirements, having a love affair with their computer right in front of you in their office, you probably won't want to listen to them either...I totally understand, but what then can happen, if **you** don't create the connection, your healthcare might suffer...you might lose more toes. Also importantly, you will be alone with your needs for help. It's not fair, it's really not your doing, but it is up to you and all of us to change this.

On a larger scale, my hope is that if many, many people resist this, and speak from their heart with their concerns, and refuse to play second fiddle to the computer and the requirements, there will be increasing charts with the required questions unanswered ("deficiencies"). At first, the analysts and regulators will do what they do, which is to put more pressure on the healthcare companies and providers to control your behavior...to use slick words and motivate you to do this the "right" way (their way), but eventually, if this can move through

our healthcare system, the bureaucracy may have to admit

defeat. Of course, they might try to regulate that too: "You will

document that you had at least 10% of charts with deficiencies

in each quarter to show that you are listening to your clients."

(Yes, that was a joke, hopefully.)

This comes at an important time in healthcare, because

there is a bright light on the horizon...more focus is being given

to what is called "Client Centered" care, which simply means

that the provider should tailor his or her approach and treatments

to what you want, not just what research and protocols might

recommend. You don't want that chemotherapy? No MRI for

you? You would rather have your blood pressure a little higher

than take a second medicine for it so you don't have to deal with

the side effects? It is your healthcare and your life, to live as you

see fit, and if the ideas in this book become a "movement" that destabilizes the rush to more and more control over what happens with your doctor at your visit, this idea and Client Centered care will fit perfectly together. After all, centering care on your desires will necessarily mean that providers will have to listen to you, not ask an endless succession of required screening questions.

I know of another woman who was having facial pain and was seen in an ER. She had a perfectly normal exam, with no evidence of a stroke, but the ER MD, after consulting a Neurologist by phone, recommended a CT scan of her head with contrast dye. The Neurologist had not seen the client, and in this case doctors, at a distance over the phone, often feel pressed to recommend lots of tests to protect themselves. The client refused the contrast, but agreed to the scan, knowing well that the contrast dye carries a small risk of serious kidney damage. Upon hearing this, the ER doctor immediately asked her to sign out "against medical advice" (AMA). That MD could have relented and at least ordered a scan without the contrast, documenting that her client refused the contrast, or she could have continued working with her client to develop care in the absence of using the scan at all and propose follow up, but the doctor's reaction was black and white, almost as if she had been insulted by the client's request.

This kind of behavior is outdated and belongs in the past. The fact is that providers, clients, healthcare systems, and the government agencies that regulate them should be working together to provide care that supports your needs and wishes, based on your life, not their ideas of who you should be or what you should do.

So please go out and make yourself heard. Make it clear that you are there to discuss what your concerns and worries and symptoms are, not what the doctor or an analyst want you to discuss. Speak up about what kind of treatment you'd like, and ask what the range of options are, knowing that often the provider will only discuss a limited set of options with you because of their own rigidity or the regulations or fears they live with. The Internet can be wonderful in this, as you can find that there may be several other ways of treating a problem than what the provider proposes, and if you come prepared, you can make this a part of the conversation.

If you meet such resistance from the provider that you don't feel you can be heard, ask for a second opinion or to switch to another provider...you cannot have good healthcare without your concerns being addressed....

You will be the only one who can change this, both for you, and hopefully, for the system as a whole.

PART TWO: PSYCHIATRY

In part two, I'd like to look at psychiatry specifically, as perhaps more than other medical specialties, the connection and communication is vital to your ability to heal. Unfortunately the history of psychiatry and psychotherapy, and its changes through this upheaval in medicine, has been parallel and I think (yes, I am biased), more profound. Connection is important through all specialties in medicine, but more so in psychiatry.

Chapter One: Connection

Somewhere, something incredible is waiting to be known.

Carl Sagan

How many of your neighbors do you know? How many of your Facebook contacts do you know? How well do you know your partner? How well do you know your children and what they are doing? How well do they know their friends or the people they've met on the Internet? Have you sat on your porch lately and talked to people walking by? Have you ever had a huge conflict over a misinterpreted text? Have you sat next to someone you loved and talked to them very little while both of your were staring at your screens?

It's an easy shot, but not a cheap one, to say we live in an increasingly disconnected world. We can increasingly feel alone, but superficially connected to many in our lives.

For much longer, however, it has been a very common human experience to feel alone, even with people close by, even before we had the number of distractions we have today...

We are born, I think, unconcerned about who we are...we are just alive. We want to crawl around and explore, eat, laugh, cry, yell, poop, and everything else that is part of life. We want to be safe, and very definitely we want to be loved. That's the hook. If we are raised with a feeling that above all we are loved for who we are and who we are becoming then we can grow up feeling connected in relationships. However, most of the time we become "domesticated" from our free spirit to a human bonsai tree...meaning that we are taught that we are lovable and will be safe **if** we act a certain way, look a certain way, talk a certain way, think a certain way, feel a certain way. We are OK

if we are a certain age or weight or color or from a particular

country or heritage or religion. To be safe and loved we create a

person for all to see who will not be attacked, who will be

admired, who apparently makes no mistakes, who won't be

criticized or punished. This person is not who we really

are...we've forgotten that person, that child who approached the

world with wonder, looking outward. We look inside and see

our fears, and think that who we really are is unworthy or worse.

If people really knew us, they wouldn't love us, or worse, we'd

be attacked...maybe even stoned to death in the town square, but

at the very least alone, poor, starving...a pitiful creature. So we

try harder to create an image for everyone...and ironically, since

it isn't really our true self, we can now be apparently connected,

even apparently intimately, and yet feel lost and alone. If we

could see the spirit that has been in us from the beginning, we would relax...and the people who also loved that true spirit would stick by us. We would find happiness in being just ourselves. We would be free again. It can feel so hopeless, though, because of what we think we are, and also our shame at what we've done to sooth the fear and aloneness...drugs, alcohol, misplaced lust and sex, hunger for power and money, violence, hatred of others...all to sooth the sense of hatred of self.

Failing, in our own minds, we then often look to others to complete us. After all, aren't we responsible for their feelings and lives (and they for ours)? We can then be furious when they don't complete us, and feel even worse about ourselves underneath.

We can discover our original selves again, and people can support us in this, but we can never find ourselves by thinking that others complete us.

This kind of aloneness has been with people for a very long time, and a lot has been written about it, and about the rediscovery of our original selves. One particularly moving poem about this rediscovery was written almost 800 years ago:

Do not be satisfied with the stories that come before you.
Unfold your own myth.

There is a candle in your heart, ready to be kindled.
There is a void in your soul, ready to be filled.
You feel it, don't you?
I want to sing like the birds sing, not worrying about
who hears or what they think.

Set your life on fire. Seek those who fan your flames

Rumi

The exploration of this idea and the process is far deeper than I can approach in this book, but I can suggest three books that have much wisdom about this process...books that taught me as much about myself and other people as the years of

medical school, psychiatry residency, and practice combined:

There Is Nothing Wrong With You by Cheri Huber (Keep It

Simple Books, 2001)

The Four Agreements by don Miguel Ruiz (Amber-Allen

Publishing, Inc., 1997)

in the MEANTIME...finding yourself and the love that you want

by Iyanla Vanzant (Simon & Schuster , 2007)

They are each from different spiritual or philosophical

points of view, but the messages they contain are amazingly

similar. They fit well together, and if you are struggling with

yourself and your relationships, they can be a turning point for

you.

In our aloneness, especially if we have no friends that we

can fully confide in, we often turn to therapists to help. This very act, aside from all the theories about how therapy works, is a statement of being unable to do it alone, and a willingness to ask someone to go through this with you, at your side.

We've discussed the importance of the alliance between a provider and a client in health care. Several studies have shown this (and you knew it all along, didn't you)! Many organizations have extensively looked at the alliance between you and your provider, and you can easily search the Internet for and see the breadth of this research. There is a common thread in their results: that more focus needs to be made on the emotional and spiritual aspects of the healing relationship. Yet we continue to focus on the intellectual aspect and the numbers. We focus on the labels, the medicines, and the prescribed treatments for each label. Psychiatry for many years was a safe haven for a healing connection to flourish, but unfortunately it also has fallen prey to the same influences that medicine in general has.

Chapter Two: The Soul of Psychiatry

We're all just walking each other home.

Ram Das

Psychiatrists and psychotherapists, like other specialists, often went into that specialty because they were fascinated by how peoples' minds worked and what could be done to help them. There is an adventure to this career, just like in medicine as a whole...each person is a whole new world, even though we often have common sufferings and joys, each person can be a new novel, a new song. It really is a privilege to listen to each person's life...and the wisdom a therapist gains from this as a provider is much greater than what they have been taught.

Psychotherapists also sometimes come from troubled backgrounds themselves, and might have been the peacemakers or the therapists for their families when younger. Just like the rest of us, they can get caught up in feeling that they are not worthy, that they are hurt (and they wonder how they can help you). Sometimes they try to reassure themselves that they are OK because of their profession: after all, if they are helping other people, they must be doing pretty good, right? Some therapists don't even recognize this in themselves, and hide themselves in the world of "My patients are to be pitied, but I am just wonderful." From your standpoint, you may feel pitied or that your therapist is condescending or aloof when this happens. With the authority that you might give to therapists, this might worsen your sense of self worth and seem to confirm your fears.

Just like the rest of us, therapists need to go through the same steps of the rediscovery of their inherent goodness, to see beyond their fears. When they've done this, their ability to connect with you becomes even more powerful, their need to see you as ill and themselves as superior can disappear, and what I've found is that their own suffering and recovery gives them the greatest ability to understand and help others, once they truly care about themselves.

This whole process of self-discovery, for both you and your therapist, occurs probably over the entirety of both of your lives. It occurs even during the visits you have, but it takes time: time for that therapist to listen to you, and to listen to himself or herself as well.

Psychiatry in the 1980s was a combination of this process and the increasingly important area of biological psychiatry.

New understanding of mental suffering and its biological causes was rapidly expanding. There was a tension between the two, with advocates of each view at times belittling the other "side." Really, it was ludicrous...if you want to understand why a car does what it does, you have to understand both the car and the driver. Some tried to mechanistically reduce all of a person's reactions to biological processes. ("What else is there?", they thought.) Ignoring the energetic, social or spiritual aspect of our existence, biology was felt to be underneath personality, decision-making, and all emotional reactions. In this conflict between these two schools of thought, biology began to win, and increasingly what the person experienced in their lives and its meaning to them became less important as a focus for intervention.

The therapist, however, who could focus and listen to you and the complex interplay of your history, events, family life, and culture, or who could balance this process and the biological aspects of your suffering, had the time to truly develop an understanding of what you were going through and help you make decisions about how to change the way you looked at yourself and others. This could allow you to discover yourself and be friends with yourself once again, and allow your relationships with others to deepen.

This took time, though, and what happened in medicine in general, happened in psychotherapy as well. Increasingly, the psychotherapists of the 1990s found that they were told that they wouldn't be paid to see their clients more than once a month (or less), even if that client needed the help. The frequency and **total** number of allowed visits dropped sharply. In private practice, we often found ourselves on the phone with people from the health insurance companies trying to convince them to allow us to see you more often than they would allow. The focus was on efficient, quick intervention, and quite expectedly, the biological aspects of your care began to take priority.

Psychiatrists especially, having MDs and being able to prescribe medicines, came under a lot of pressure to target depression for example, and use a medication to treat it, and have follow up visits focused on the side effects and response to the medicine.

From your standpoint, **your** work life was getting busier as well (as our nation's productivity climbed rapidly to eventually become one of the highest in the world today, despite the minimum wage, inflation adjusted, now being 25% lower).

When **you** had little time to see someone to try and sort out what was going wrong, getting a pill to fix it seemed like the easiest, most efficient solution. You didn't have to miss much work, and you also didn't really have to talk about a lot of the painful parts of your life.

I really lost track during this period of how many people I tried medicine after medicine for their depression (the most common problem treated), sometimes with partial or no relief, only to find later that the need for a medicine disappeared when that client came to a new understanding of themselves, often with a change of job, or a relationship, or lifestyle. This happened sometimes on its own, as we didn't have the time to explore this much in our visits...but I fear for a lot of others it didn't happen at all, so the medicine quests continued with all the inherent risks and side effects.

As the number of visits allowed dropped, correspondingly, even in a private practice the number of people the therapists were providing care to increased. The depth of the understanding was more superficial, and the limited stories you told us unfortunately started to run together (after all, we were really only getting a superficial sketch of what was happening). Just as in other specialties, it became easy to confuse one client with another. How would this feel to to you? Again, you could feel unimportant and increasingly alone...just what we didn't want. The soul of the profession was poisoned.

Chapter Three: Don't Sit Down

Time is a created thing. To say 'I don't have time' is like saying 'I don't want to.'
Lao Tzu

As the degradation of the therapeutic relationship continued, clients grew increasingly frustrated. Therapists themselves were frustrated, but faced with increasing difficulty getting paid, began to work for systems of care who were under the gun as well. Adding to this mess was the longstanding, systemic bigotry against mental health services. Medicare during this period, for example, reimbursed private practice psychotherapy providers 50% for the fees that Medicare felt reasonable, and 80% for other medical specialties. There has always been a devaluing of things psychiatric, as if it were frivolous and just pandering to "whiners," not realizing that it is our experience of ourselves and life that often creates the greatest hell for us, and leads us to poor self care and decisions that severely worsen our overall health. This bigotry exists in health care, among providers, in governmental agencies, and in fact is deep in our society.

Now transfixed with the computer, and then overwhelmed with increasingly complex regulations--the same complex regulations that I touched on in part one, therapists were spending less and less time trying to understand their clients. (They were also not exempted from asking all the required questions, for example, about weight, exercise, smoking, etc., because of their specialty.) Medicines were becoming more important. Group therapy, which is very powerful but overwhelms and puts off many who are convinced they are sickened inside, and who don't want to talk about their fears in front of a group, became the increasing mode of treatment.

Many times I heard stories like this: "He didn't even look at me, he just asked me a bunch of questions and wrote me a prescription." "She never looked up from her computer, she just typed the whole time." "I can't even get in to see him, and he doesn't answer my questions in my e mails." "She told me to quit complaining and take responsibility for my life and that she couldn't help me." (Please don't get me wrong--it is vital that you take responsibility for your life, but it is an enormous blessing to have someone to help you in this quest.) I've heard of people who had been traumatized and sent to a group, with little follow up to build trust and a place that felt safe to talk. The gallows humor joke was that clients shouldn't even sit down...there was no time for that.

Increasingly, emphasis was put on labeling the client for insurance purposes (who then could be in essence be written off and simplified, a cartoon of who they really are), and putting them in a fairly rigid path of care, number of visits, and specified medications for the label they had.

Medicines themselves have shown themselves to be increasingly dangerous to use, and the glowing reports of the drug companies as to their effectiveness were often found to be very inflated. Some studies have even suggested that antidepressants aren't much better than placebos in treating depression. The number of potentially serious side effects has grown, which is frightening for you and a minefield for the prescriber. I certainly have seen a lot of people for whom medicines were life saving, but the percentage of improvement in people overall has often not been what was at first presented.

Underneath this now, there is no time for therapists to take the time to think about these things and systemic problems much, but just to push on and do the best they can. The regulators and analysts who have demanded that their requirements be fulfilled will also, along with health insurance companies and other providers, blame the provider for mistakes in care. Please don't think this is just sour grapes on my part--I was lucky enough that I was never sued in my career, but the threat of criticism and consequences is always there, and more importantly, always there is the provider's fear that something will happen to one of their clients: suicide, a fatal or severe drug reaction, or other bad result.

The burn out rate for doctors in psychiatry stands at 38%, not the worst, (it ranges up to 50% plus for other specialties and general practice doctors), but a far cry from the amazing experience it used to be for most therapists and clients.

The remedy remains the same, and unfortunately it still relies on you speaking up. The time you have with a therapist is yours, and you have a right to be heard. You have a right to ask for individual, one on one care, at least for the first several visits, to be seen more often, to be understood and known for more than your label and your current medication trial. You may not be able to be seen weekly, but you should be able to be seen more often than is usual today.

There may be a lot of push back from some providers, and underneath this they may feel pressured, exhausted, angry, trapped. What you may hear are things like: "Now Ms. X, we can help a lot of people with our classes and groups, and I'd really like you to give this a try...what are your concerns about this?"

My suggestion to this and other very crafted replies by your provider is to reply with something like: "I'm willing to think about that in the future, but for now I feel fearful, lost, alone, and I need to have a trusting relationship with you first; to know I can rely on you to listen and see me regularly through this whole thing. I don't yet feel comfortable going to classes and groups." "I don't think seeing me months from now or just giving me a medicine is right for me." Or: " I know you're very busy, but I'd rather see you by myself for awhile before I start all the other treatments you'd like."

Again, the point is not to attack the provider, but to speak from your heart, as no one can truly take that away from you. You may feel unworthy inside, angry, or fearful, but if your voice is shaking and your hands trembling, speak up from your heart and say it anyway. If your provider refuses to bend, ask for another until you find one willing to develop that trust with you.

You can still go to groups one day and gain all the wonderful help that provides; you can go to classes to learn many valuable things about what you're going through, but first you need that close trusting alliance. Whatever you do, don't give up. Insist that you need to be seen. You may be told something to the effect of: "Well, you didn't click with provider X, so we won't be able to get you in for another 3 weeks." Speak from your heart, tell the person you're talking to that this isn't acceptable, and if they resist, ask to speak to the head of their clinic. It may help to have someone you trust sitting with you for strength. You are not wrong to ask for help, you are not weak, you are human. You, or someone else is paying for this care and **you deserve it.**

Chapter Four: Consequences

He was such a nice, quiet kid

(Said by many.)

The lack of mental health care, devalued, underfunded, often unavailable to people with severe suffering, is harming our society.

The figures are too well known and sad:

• About half of people in prison have a mental disorder, and their rate of return to prison is higher than other prisoners. I can tell you by experience that, while there are some good Psychiatrists in the prison system, often the Psychiatric care is poor or spotty. Medications get discontinued, diagnoses dismissed (at times after one visit with the new provider). The client can come out in worse shape, with their symptoms uncontrolled.

- Most of the time, prisoners with mental illnesses are not in prison for violent crimes (they more often are the victims of violent crimes). They are often imprisoned for drug abuse or other non-violent crimes. Again, drugs are a quick way out of the suffering of mental disorders, and drug use crimes make up for a large part of our prison population.

- More than 1/5th of the homeless have severe mental disorders, and this of course, without help, worsens the hope of getting out of their horrible situation.

- Over 30% of Veterans have at least one mental disorder, and many of the homeless are veterans.

What has not been born out by statistics is a clear association between violence and mental disorders, and in fact people with diagnosed mental disorders are **less likely** to commit violent crimes. However, this speaks to the point that people without a "diagnosis" can kill. What is almost certainly true is that some of the gun violence might have been prevented by mental health care and a more connected society than the one we have. Our family dynamics have changed over the years to favor isolated small groups in place of an extended family. With increasing alienation from each other, mental health services become even more needed to provide the support that a family, a community, and a culture used to provide.

Violence is almost certainly built into all of us, and I do feel that the more connected we are to each other, the less likely we are to kill each other. It also speaks to the availability of guns to what we consider normal citizens. It often seems that people with no known mental illness kill, but again, how much of a part does the hell that we can all create inside for ourselves play in this? While mental illness labels may be applied to a fraction of our population, mental **suffering** and drug use could be underlying most of the violence in our culture. It could be that if therapy could help people to truly care for themselves, they wouldn't turn to drugs and wouldn't kill others to ease their own suffering.

PART THREE:

FINAL THOUGHTS

AND PRAYER

Our country, our world, desperately needs compassionate connection and compassionate healthcare.

No one should have to go to sleep at night fearing that something will happen to them or their partner/spouse, parents, children or loved ones that won't be helped by the caring of others, and by caring providers. The most heartbreaking moments in my career were when someone walked out of my office, unable to return because they no longer had healthcare. At other times, when I worked for a county agency that did help those without insurance, it was also heartbreaking to try and get a specialist to see my client, as often no one would see them because they didn't belong to their healthcare group or plan, or they would be paid little or nothing.

Equally as tragic, though, is having healthcare, but feeling like you don't exist in that office...that you were just work, an annoyance, or more subtly, not heard or seen so that you may be left with the worry that there is something very wrong with you physically that the doctor missed, leaving you alone and on your own with your fears. It is also tragic that you can feel trapped by your fears, not about your body, but of whom you fear you are, instead of rediscovering who you truly are.

I pray that healthcare is available for everyone one day, and that it finds its heart again in the profound connection of two human beings facing a problem together.

EPILOGUE

I was finishing rewriting this book for about the fifth time, and finding out just how much I'd forgotten about grammar and punctuation, when my wife and I took time off to take one of her relatives to an MD appointment.

The doctor was a bit late, a bit rushed, but amazingly, introduced himself, shook our hands, sat and looked at each of us while he was talking, and answered all of our questions with understanding. He focused on each of us in turn. He had a **conversation** with us. At the end of the visit, my in-law was feeling better and more hopeful, and you could see this in his energy and spirit.

I was impressed--this doctor seemed to be back about ten or fifteen years in time. I'm a little slow visually at times, but I finally noticed that in his hands was a paper chart. My wife asked him about this when we were leaving the room. " Yeah, in three weeks we're switching to a computerized chart, and I'm not looking forward to it, because I figure my back is going to be toward the patient, and I'll be typing into the computer," he said.

I didn't say anything. I hope that he and the people seeing him enjoy the time together now and over the next three weeks.

NOTES

PART ONE: MEDICINE

CHAPTER ONE: IT WAS ALWAYS ABOUT THE MONEY

1).   *Sicko* (movie) 2007, Director: Michael Moore

CHAPTER TWO: THE MACHINES AND THEIR

ATTENDANTS

2).   *Moneyball* (movie) 2011, Director Bennett Miller, and

based on the book *Moneyball: The Art of Winning an Unfair*

Game by Michael Lewis (2003, W.W. Norton and Co.)

CHAPTER THREE: WHO ARE THE ANALYSTS?

3). "Building Healthcare Delivery Around Quality:

Implementing the National Quality Strategy"

(Kate Goodrich, MD, MHS; Nancy J. Wilson, MD, MPH

February 26th, 2014, Supported by the **Centers for Medicare**

& Medicaid Services, a U.S. Department of Health and Human

Services, published on the website "Medscape"

www.medscape.com)

4). *Gallipoli (*movie) 1981, director Peter Weir

5). From the CMS website on July 8th, 2015:

https://www.cms.gov/Regulations-and-

Guidance/Legislation/EHRIncentivePrograms/downloads/EP-

MU-TOC.pdf

CHAPTER FOUR: THE SPIRIT OF CARING UNDER

ASSAULT

6).   "Physician Burnout: It Just Keeps Getting Worse" (Carol

Peckham January 26th, 2015 published on the website

Medscape www.medscape.com)